Conquering Breast Cancer

A Guide to Prevention and Recovery.

Dr Scott Mendoza

Table Of Contents

Title: Conquering Breast Cancer: A Guide to Prevention and Recovery

INTRODUCTION

"Conquering Breast Cancer: A Guide to Prevention and Recovery" is a beacon of knowledge, empathy, and empowerment in the face of a daunting diagnosis. This comprehensive and compassionate resource is designed to serve as a steadfast companion for individuals, families, and caregivers navigating the intricate terrain of breast cancer. From demystifying the science behind the disease to equipping readers with practical tools for prevention, treatment, and holistic recovery, this book stands as a testament to resilience, hope, and the indomitable human spirit.

From one chapter to the next, "Conquering Breast Cancer" probes into the multifaceted landscape of this complex illness, illuminating key concepts, strategies, and insights essential for forging a path to wellness. It begins by unraveling the enigma of breast cancer, offering a clear understanding of its biological underpinnings, risk factors, and the pivotal role of early detection. With heartfelt emphasis on preventive measures, the book presents proactive lifestyle modifications, advocating for the transformative power of nutrition, exercise, stress management, and environmental awareness in reducing risk and enhancing overall health.

When we talk about breast cancer treatment, the book remains an unwavering guide, dissecting the array of options available to patients. From surgical considerations to the nuances of chemotherapy, radiation therapy, and cutting-edge targeted and immunotherapies, it extends a reassuring hand, offering clarity, encouraging questions, and laying the foundation for informed decision-making.

Beyond conventional methods, "Conquering Breast Cancer" wholeheartedly embraces integrative approaches to healing, championing the synergy of complementary and alternative medicine, mind-body practices, and holistic wellness in fostering resilience and fortifying the body's innate capacity for recovery.

Yet, the book is not confined to the physical aspects of the disease. It bravely and sensitively navigates the emotional and mental terrain, tending to the profound impact of a breast cancer diagnosis on the psyche. Offering solace in shared experiences, it guides readers through the ebbs and flows of emotion, instilling hope, and providing actionable strategies for maintaining mental well-being. Drawing strength from personal narratives and professional insights, it underscores the pivotal importance of a robust support system and the accessibility of mental health resources in fostering inner fortitude and emotional equilibrium.

Even as treatment concludes, this book gracefully
extends its embrace, acknowledging the phase of
recovery and transition. It illuminates the contours of
survivorship, navigating the labyrinth of follow-up care,
redefining notions of body image, and nurturing
enduring resilience and vitality. Bolstered by a reservoir
of practical advice and inspirational tales of triumph, it
urges readers to envision a fulfilling life beyond cancer,
resonating with the mantra of perseverance and the
echo of new beginnings.

Lastly, this book champions not only personal
empowerment but societal advocacy, boldly confronting
stigmatization and misinformation, and advocating for
heightened awareness, improved policies, and amplified
funding to redefine the breast cancer landscape. It
celebrates the unassailable human spirit, amplifying the
voices of survivors, caregivers, and advocates, and
uniting readers in a tapestry of shared humanity and
unwavering hope.

In its essence, "Conquering Breast Cancer" transcends
the boundaries of a mere guidebook; it is a manifesto of
resilience, a testament to empowerment, and a beacon
of unwavering hope. It invites readers to embark on a
journey of knowledge, healing, and fortitude, honoring
the sacred contract between information and inspiration,
between science and the soul. With Every page turned,
it kindles a spark of optimism, illuminating the path

towards a future defined not by fear, but by the triumph of the human spirit over adversity.

Chapter 1: Understanding Breast Cancer

1.1 What is Breast Cancer

Breast cancer is a complex disease characterized by the uncontrolled growth of abnormal cells in the breast tissue. These cells have the potential to invade surrounding tissues and can spread to other parts of the body, leading to the formation of secondary tumors, a process known as metastasis.
Understanding the fundamental nature of breast cancer is essential in order to comprehend its impact, take proactive steps for prevention, and effectively engage in treatment and recovery.

Fundamentally, breast cancer originates from genetic mutations that prompt normal breast cells to undergo unregulated growth. These mutations can occur due to a variety of factors, including inherited genetic predispositions, environmental influences, and hormonal imbalances. While not all breast cancers are linked to genetic factors, an individual's genetic makeup can significantly influence their susceptibility to the disease.

When discussing breast cancer, it's crucial to recognize the various types and subtypes that exist, each with distinct characteristics and varying implications for treatment and prognosis. For instance, ductal carcinoma in situ (DCIS) and invasive ductal carcinoma are among the more common forms, while lobular carcinoma in situ (LCIS) and invasive lobular carcinoma represent other subtypes. Additionally, certain breast cancers are defined by the absence of hormone receptors or HER2 protein expression, which can significantly impact treatment strategies and outcomes.

Early detection plays an important role in addressing breast cancer effectively. Screening methods, such as mammography, clinical breast exams, and self-examination techniques, are critical in detecting abnormalities at an early, more treatable stage. Once an abnormality is identified, diagnostic procedures, including biopsies and pathological analysis, are essential for confirming the presence of cancer and gaining insights into its specific characteristics, thus guiding subsequent treatment decisions.

Furthermore, understanding the risk factors associated with breast cancer is paramount in formulating prevention strategies. While some risk factors, such as age and genetic predisposition, are beyond an individual's control, lifestyle choices, including diet, physical activity, and alcohol consumption, can significantly influence one's risk profile. Educating individuals on these modifiable risk factors empowers them to make informed decisions and adopt proactive measures to reduce their susceptibility to the disease.

In conclusion, a comprehensive understanding of breast cancer encompasses its biological mechanisms, the diverse array of subtypes, the importance of early detection, and modifiable risk factors. Equipping individuals with this knowledge fosters a proactive stance in prevention, underscores the significance of regular screenings, and empowers informed decision-making in the pursuit of optimal breast health.

1.2 Risk Factors and Proactive Prevention Strategies

Breast Cancer Risk Factors:

Breast cancer is influenced by a multitude of risk factors, some of which are beyond individual control, while others can be modified through proactive measures.

Genetic predisposition and family history play a significant role, with inherited mutations in genes such as BRCA1 and BRCA2 increasing the likelihood of developing the disease.

Additionally, age is a crucial factor, as the risk of breast cancer rises as individuals grow older, particularly after menopause.

Hormonal influences, such as early menstruation, late menopause, and prolonged use of hormone replacement therapy, also contribute to heightened susceptibility.

Other non-modifiable risk factors include certain benign breast conditions, previous chest radiation, and personal history of breast cancer or high-risk lesions.

Exclusive Prevention Strategies:

1. **Genetic Counseling and Testing**: For individuals with a strong family history of breast cancer, genetic counseling and testing can provide valuable insights, enabling informed decisions about risk management and preventative measures.

2. **Lifestyle Modifications**: Adopting a healthy lifestyle can significantly impact breast cancer risk. Engaging in regular physical activity, maintaining a balanced diet rich in fruits, vegetables, and whole grains, limiting alcohol consumption, and avoiding tobacco products are all conducive to reducing risk.

3. **Hormonal Management**: Minimizing exposure to hormonal influences, such as avoiding unnecessary hormone replacement therapy and discussing alternative options with healthcare providers, can mitigate risk.

4. **Breastfeeding:** For women who are able to breastfeed, doing so may offer protective benefits against breast cancer. Learning about the potential advantages and considering breastfeeding as a natural preventative measure can be beneficial.

5. **Vigilant Monitoring and Screening**: Adhering to recommended screening guidelines, such as regular mammograms and clinical breast exams, fosters early detection, thereby maximizing treatment options and improving outcomes.

6. **Awareness and Education**: Promoting breast health awareness and educating individuals about the significance of self-examinations and early detection is pivotal. Empowering individuals to recognize changes in their breast tissue and seek prompt medical attention enhances proactive engagement in their health journey.

Ultimately, comprehending the interplay of risk factors associated with breast cancer equips individuals with the knowledge necessary to implement effective prevention strategies. By advocating for genetic counseling, fostering a health-conscious lifestyle, being mindful of hormonal influences, embracing breastfeeding, adhering to screening protocols, and enhancing breast health awareness, individuals can meaningfully reduce their susceptibility to this complex disease, thus ushering in a culture of proactive engagement and empowerment in the quest for optimal breast health.

1.3. Exploring the Diverse Types of Breast Cancer and Their Unique Characteristics

Breast cancer encompasses a spectrum of distinct types, each characterized by specific biological features, behaviors, and implications for treatment. Understanding the nuances of these variations is crucial in guiding tailored approaches to diagnosis, management, and care.

1. Ductal Carcinoma In Situ (DCIS):
· DCIS represents a non-invasive form of breast cancer, where abnormal cells are confined to the milk ducts. While not invasive, if left untreated, DCIS can potentially progress to invasive cancer. Detection and early intervention are critical in addressing this type of breast cancer.

2. **Invasive Ductal Carcinoma (IDC):**

This is the most common type of breast cancer, characterized by cancer cells that invade surrounding breast tissue outside the ducts. IDC can present with diverse growth patterns, contributing to variations in prognosis and treatment strategies.

3. **Lobular Carcinoma In Situ (LCIS):**

LCIS involves abnormal cell growth within the lobules of the breast, often considered a marker indicating an increased risk of developing invasive cancer in either breast.

4. **Invasive Lobular Carcinoma (ILC):**

ILC originates in the lobules and has the potential to spread beyond the breast to other parts of the body. It is known for its unique growth patterns, which can pose challenges in detection through imaging techniques.

5. **Triple-Negative Breast Cancer (TNBC):**

TNBC lacks estrogen, progesterone, and HER2 receptor expression, making it unresponsive to hormonal and HER2-targeted therapies. This subtype tends to be more aggressive and is associated with a poorer prognosis.

6. **Hormone Receptor-Positive Breast Cancer:**

This subtype is characterized by the presence of hormone receptors, specifically estrogen and/or progesterone. Targeting these receptors through hormone-based therapies forms the cornerstone of treatment for this type of breast cancer.

7. HER2-Positive Breast Cancer:
HER2-positive breast cancer cells overexpress the HER2 protein, contributing to aggressive tumor growth. Targeted therapies aimed at HER2 receptors have revolutionized the management of this subtype, significantly improving outcomes.

8. Inflammatory Breast Cancer:
This rare and aggressive type of breast cancer often presents with redness, swelling, and warmth in the breast, resembling an inflammation. It necessitates prompt and comprehensive treatment due to its rapid progression.

Understanding the distinctive characteristics of each breast cancer subtype is pivotal in guiding personalized treatment strategies, optimizing patient outcomes, and advancing research initiatives. By acknowledging the diverse nature of breast cancer and tailoring interventions to individual requirements, healthcare providers can navigate this complex landscape with precision and compassion, ultimately enhancing the quality of care and fostering hope for those affected by this pervasive disease.

1.4 Early Detection and Diagnosis: The Critical Imperative for Combatting Breast Cancer

The significance of early detection and diagnosis in the realm of breast cancer cannot be overstated, as it represents a pivotal determinant in patient outcomes, treatment efficacy, and overall prognosis. Incorporating a multifaceted approach encompassing education, screening interventions, and proactive health management is fundamental in empowering individuals and healthcare professionals alike to confront this complex disease with precision and fortitude.

1. Enhanced Treatment Efficacy:
Early detection of breast cancer significantly enhances the range of treatment options available to patients, enabling more conservative and potentially curative interventions. This not only contributes to improved survival rates but also minimizes the need for extensive, invasive procedures, translating to a higher quality of life for afflicted individuals.

2. Reduced Mortality Rates:
Timely detection and diagnosis play a pivotal role in mitigating mortality rates associated with breast cancer. By identifying malignancies at an early stage, the potential for effective treatment and favorable long-term outcomes is substantially amplified, offering renewed hope and vitality to those affected.

3. **Facilitated Personalized Care**:
Early diagnostic insights empower healthcare providers to tailor treatment regimens to individual patient profiles, considering factors such as tumor characteristics, genetic predispositions, and overall health status. This personalized approach fosters precision medicine, optimizing therapeutic efficacy while minimizing unnecessary side effects.

4. **Minimized Disease Progression:**
Early identification of breast cancer affords the opportunity to address the disease while it is localized, curtailing the likelihood of metastasis and its associated complications. Proactive vigilance and swift intervention are paramount in impeding disease progression and preserving long-term health.

5. **Enhanced Psychosocial Well-being**:
Timely detection averts the emotional burden and distress of facing advanced or metastatic stages of breast cancer, offering patients and their families a clearer path forward and a renewed sense of agency in their health journey.

6. **Cost-Efficient Interventions:**
Early detection and diagnosis lead to more cost-effective treatments, as they decrease the necessity for extensive surgeries, prolonged hospitalizations, and intensive therapeutic interventions. By allocating resources most

efficiently, healthcare systems can better address the overarching needs of all patients.

Comprehensive and compassionate education and awareness initiatives, combined with accessible screening modalities, serve as the cornerstone for promoting early detection and diagnosis of breast cancer.
Empowering individuals to recognize the significance of regular self-examinations, clinical assessments, and imaging studies fosters proactive engagement and a steadfast commitment to prioritizing one's health. Together, these endeavors forge a collective resolve to confront breast cancer with unwavering persistence, driving forward a paradigm of early detection and diagnosis as the linchpin in our collective endeavor to enhance the well-being of individuals and communities affected by this pervasive disease.

Chapter 2. Lifestyle Changes and Prevention .

2.1 Dietary Strategies for Breast Cancer Prevention

Crafting a robust defense against breast cancer extends beyond medical interventions, encompassing the profound impact of dietary choices and nutritional patterns. Nurturing a health-conscious lifestyle rooted in wholesome, nourishing foods and mindful dietary practices constitutes a cornerstone in fortifying the body's resilience against this complex disease.

1. **Embrace Plant-Based Diversity**:
Prioritize a plant-forward dietary framework, rich in an array of colorful fruits, vegetables, legumes, and whole grains. The diverse phytonutrients, vitamins, and antioxidants present in these foods exert a protective influence, bolstering the body's natural defense mechanisms and mitigating cellular damage.

2. **Opt for Lean Protein Sources**:
Lean sources of protein, such as fish, poultry, legumes, and tofu, provide essential amino acids while moderating the intake of saturated fats commonly found

in red and processed meats. Fish, in particular, offers omega-3 fatty acids, conferring anti-inflammatory and heart-healthy benefits.

3. Cultivate Healthy Fats:
Favor healthy fats derived from sources like avocados, nuts, seeds, and olive oil, as they furnish essential fatty acids and bioactive compounds linked to reduced inflammation and improved cardiovascular health. Steering clear of trans fats and minimizing saturated fat intake contributes to overall well-being.

4. Limit Refined Sugars and Processed Foods:
Minimize the consumption of sugary beverages, refined carbohydrates, and heavily processed foods, as excessive sugar and refined components can disrupt metabolic balance and fuel oxidative stress within the body.

5. Moderate Alcohol Consumption:
Exercise prudence in alcohol consumption, as excessive intake is associated with an elevated risk of breast cancer. Limiting alcohol consumption to moderate or abstaining entirely is advisable for those seeking to proactively manage their health.

6. Maintain a Healthy Weight:
Strive towards achieving and maintaining a healthy body weight through a balanced diet and regular physical activity. Adipose tissue serves as a reservoir for

estrogen production, and elevated estrogen levels can heighten breast cancer risk, making weight management a pivotal aspect of prevention.

7. Stay Hydrated:
Adequate hydration is indispensable in promoting cellular health and metabolic function. Choosing water as the primary beverage and limiting sugary drinks and excessive caffeine fosters optimal hydration and overall well-being.

8. Embrace Mindful Eating Practices:
Cultivate an awareness of portion sizes, mindful eating, and a balanced approach to nourishment. Attuning to the body's natural cues and savoring meals mindfully can promote satiety and a harmonious relationship with food.

Curating a nutritionally sound and conscientious dietary landscape plays an instrumental role in fortifying the body's inherent defenses against breast cancer and cultivating holistic well-being. By embracing the vitality of plant-centric nutrition, balanced protein choices, healthy fats, and prudent lifestyle habits, individuals embark on a transformative journey towards proactive health preservation, imbuing each meal with the power to act as a shield against the encroachment of disease while fostering enduring vitality and resilience.

2.2. The Transformative Impact of Exercise in Breast Cancer Prevention and Recovery

Exercise and physical activity constitute a profound and transformative force in the prevention and recovery from breast cancer, wielding a multitude of benefits that intersect with physical, emotional, and psychological well-being. By embarking on a journey of movement and mindful physical engagement, individuals harness the power of exercise as a formidable ally in fortifying the body's resilience against the onset of breast cancer and as a catalyst in bolstering recovery pathways post-diagnosis and treatment.

Prevention Through Movement:
Regular physical activity serves as a key element in breast cancer prevention, conferring a spectrum of advantages that mitigate risk factors and nurture overall health:

- **Modulating Hormonal Balance**: Exercise plays a pivotal role in regulating hormonal levels, particularly estrogen, which can impact breast cancer development. By promoting hormonal equilibrium, physical activity serves as a protective measure against hormonal-driven breast malignancies.

- **Facilitating Weight Management**: Sustaining a healthy body weight through exercise regulates adipose tissue composition, contributing to a reduced risk of developing breast cancer, as excess adiposity correlates with heightened cancer susceptibility.

- Enhancing Immune Function: Physical activity nurtures a robust immune response, fortifying the body's capacity to identify and mitigate abnormal cell growth, thereby exerting a preventive influence against malignant transformations.

Recovery and Rehabilitation:
Following a breast cancer diagnosis, the integration of tailored exercise and physical activity regimens assumes a pivotal role in fostering recovery, rehabilitative progress, and overall well-being:

- Mitigating Treatment Side Effects: Exercise aids in mitigating the adverse effects of cancer treatments, such as fatigue, muscle deconditioning, and emotional distress, fostering a renewed sense of vitality and endurance.

- Promoting Lymphatic Circulation: Physical activity, including movements that engage the upper body, supports lymphatic flow, reducing the risk of lymphedema and enhancing postoperative recovery for breast cancer survivors.

- Nurturing Emotional Resilience: Engaging in regular physical activity cultivates a sense of empowerment, resilience, and emotional well-being, constituting a steadfast pillar in the holistic recovery journey post-treatment.

In embracing the transformative potential of exercise and physical activity, individuals confront breast cancer with an indomitable spirit and a proactive commitment to nurturing their health. By harnessing the vitality of movement as a gateway to prevention and recovery, they instill within themselves a profound sense of agency, resilience, and enduring well-being, transcending the confines of illness to embrace a landscape empowered by vitality and fortitude.

2.3. Stress management and emotional well-being play vital roles in preventing and aiding recovery from breast cancer.

When faced with a cancer diagnosis, individuals often experience an overwhelming array of emotions, including fear, anxiety, and sadness. These emotions, if left unaddressed, can contribute to increased stress levels, potentially impacting the body's ability to heal and recover. Therefore, maintaining emotional balance and managing stress are essential components of a comprehensive approach to breast cancer prevention and recovery.

In the context of prevention, stress management techniques such as mindfulness meditation, yoga, and deep breathing exercises can help reduce the impact of chronic stress on the body. Chronic stress can weaken the immune system and create an internal environment that is conducive to the growth of cancer cells. By incorporating stress-reducing practices into daily life, individuals can bolster their body's natural defenses, thereby reducing the likelihood of developing breast cancer.

For those undergoing treatment or in the process of recovery, emotional well-being becomes even more crucial. Managing the emotional rollercoaster that comes with a cancer diagnosis involves cultivating a support network, seeking professional therapy or counseling, and engaging in activities that promote joy and relaxation. These measures not only contribute to mental and emotional resilience but also positively influence physical health and the body's ability to respond to treatment.

Furthermore, emotional well-being and stress management can aid in mitigating the negative side effects of treatment, such as fatigue, nausea, and pain. Individuals who actively address their emotional well-being often experience improved treatment outcomes and a better quality of life during and after the recovery process.

In conclusion, prioritizing stress management and emotional well-being is integral to both preventing and recovering from breast cancer. By adopting holistic approaches that address the mind as well as the body, individuals can empower themselves to navigate the challenges of breast cancer with resilience, positivity, and strength. This comprehensive approach not only supports the body's natural healing processes but also enhances overall well-being, contributing to a higher quality of life throughout the cancer journey.

1. **Endocrine Disrupting Chemicals** (EDCs): Numerous environmental pollutants, such as bisphenol A (BPA), phthalates, and certain pesticides, have been identified as EDCs. These compounds can mimic or interfere with the body's hormonal signaling pathways, potentially increasing the risk of breast cancer. Exploring the sources and potential exposure routes to these substances can help readers make informed choices about reducing their contact with such chemicals.

2. **Radiation Exposure**: Ionizing radiation, whether from medical imaging procedures, occupational exposure, or environmental sources (e.g., radon), has been linked to an increased risk of breast cancer. Understanding the potential risks associated with radiation exposure and the importance of minimizing unnecessary exposure is

crucial for readers, especially those in high-risk
professions or regions with elevated natural radiation
levels.

3. **Lifestyle and Diet**: The impact of lifestyle and dietary
choices on breast cancer risk cannot be overlooked.
Readers can benefit from learning about the potential
influence of factors such as alcohol consumption,
obesity, and the consumption of processed foods or a
high-fat diet. Understanding how these factors interact
with genetic predispositions can empower individuals to
make positive changes and mitigate their risk.

4. **Air and Water Pollution**: Emerging research
suggests that environmental pollutants in the air and
water may play a role in breast cancer development.
Investigating the sources of these pollutants, their
potential impact on breast cancer risk, and advocating
for policies that promote clean air and water can be of
significant interest to readers concerned about
environmental factors.

5. **The Built Environment**: Urban planning, industrial
activities, and residential proximity to known sources of
environmental contamination can all impact breast
cancer risk. Exploring how the built environment affects
exposure to potential carcinogens and advocating for
community and urban design that minimizes such risks
is an important aspect for concerned readers.

By looking into these environmental factors and their impact on breast cancer, readers can gain a more comprehensive understanding of the interconnectedness between human health and the environment. This knowledge can empower individuals to make informed decisions, advocate for policy changes, and support initiatives aimed at reducing environmental factors that contribute to breast cancer incidence.

Chapter 3: Treatment Options and Strategies

3.1 Surgery: Mastectomy vs. Lumpectomy

When it comes to treating breast cancer, surgical intervention is often a critical component of a patient's journey.

The decision between mastectomy and lumpectomy, two primary surgical options, is a pivotal point in the treatment process. Here's indispensable information one need at hand for considering these options:

Mastectomy:

Mastectomy involves the surgical removal of the entire breast. This procedure is further categorized into different types, including total (simple) mastectomy, modified radical mastectomy, and skin-sparing mastectomy. In cases where the cancer is extensive, aggressive, or presents in multiple areas of the breast, mastectomy may be recommended. It provides a comprehensive approach to removing affected tissue and can be a proactive measure to prevent the potential spread or recurrence of cancer in the breast.

Lumpectomy (Breast-Conserving Surgery):

Contrastingly, lumpectomy, also known as breast-conserving surgery, involves the removal of the tumor and a portion of surrounding healthy tissue, leaving the majority of the breast intact. This approach is often preferred when the cancer is localized and small in size, allowing for less invasive treatment while preserving the natural appearance of the breast. Following a lumpectomy, radiation therapy is typically recommended to target any remaining cancer cells in the breast.

Decision-Making Factors:

It must be understood that the choice between mastectomy and lumpectomy is not solely based on medical necessity; it also involves personal preferences, emotional well-being, and the potential impact on body image. Factors such as the size and location of the tumor, the individual's overall health, genetic predispositions, and the potential need for additional treatments (e.g., radiation therapy) all come into play. Therefore, it is crucial for patients to engage in thorough discussions with their healthcare providers to weigh the pros and cons of each option based on their unique circumstances.

In summary, the decision between mastectomy and lumpectomy is a deeply personal one, influenced not

only by medical considerations but also by the individual's values and emotional well-being.
 Comprehensive information about these surgical options equips patient to make informed decisions and actively participate in the treatment planning process, ensuring that her chosen approach aligns with heir overall well-being and long-term quality of life.

3.2 Chemotherapy: Understanding the Process and Side Effects

Chemotherapy is a cornerstone of cancer treatment, including breast cancer. Providing readers with a deep understanding of the process and potential side effects is crucial for anyone considering or undergoing this form of treatment.

Understanding the Process:

Chemotherapy involves the use of powerful medications to destroy fast-growing cancer cells. These medications can be administered orally, intravenously, or through injections.
For breast cancer, chemotherapy may be recommended before surgery to shrink the tumor (neoadjuvant therapy), or after surgery to eliminate any remaining

cancer cells (adjuvant therapy). We should understand that chemotherapy is often delivered in cycles, allowing the body time to recover between treatments.

Side Effects:

Enlightenment about potential side effects is essential for preparing the patients for the challenges they may face during chemotherapy. Common side effects include nausea, vomiting, hair loss, fatigue, increased susceptibility to infections, and changes in blood cell counts.
Furthermore, chemotherapy can affect fertility in both men and women, and it may lead to early menopause in some cases. These information about these potential side effects empowers the patient to anticipate and cope with the physical and emotional impact of treatment.

Managing Side Effects:

Equipping readers with strategies to manage or mitigate side effects is paramount. This includes discussing the potential role of anti-nausea medications, dietary adjustments, physical activity, and emotional support. Additionally, informing readers about the importance of close communication with their healthcare team regarding any side effects they experience is crucial to ensure timely interventions and adjustments to the treatment plan.

In conclusion, by providing comprehensive information on the chemotherapy process and its potential side effects, readers are better prepared to navigate this form of treatment. Empowering them with knowledge about what to expect and how to manage potential side effects fosters a sense of control and resilience during what can be a challenging phase of their cancer journey. This understanding can lead to improved adherence to treatment, better quality of life during chemotherapy, and an enhanced overall treatment experience.

3.3. Radiation Therapy : Benefits and Risks.

Radiation therapy stands as a crucial pillar in the comprehensive treatment of various cancers, including breast cancer. Probing into the benefits and risks of this therapeutic modality equips you with essential knowledge for making informed decisions and confidently navigating their treatment journey.

Benefits:

Radiation therapy offers a range of benefits essential for readers to comprehend fully. By delivering targeted doses of radiation to cancer-affected areas, this treatment aims to destroy lingering cancer cells following surgery or, in some cases, to shrink tumors before surgical intervention. It plays a pivotal role in reducing the risk of cancer recurrence, thus enhancing long-term outcomes for patients. Furthermore, readers should understand the potential for palliative radiation therapy, which can alleviate symptoms and improve the quality of life for individuals with advanced breast cancer.

Risks:

The discussion of radiation therapy's risks is equally vital. You should be informed about potential acute side effects, such as skin irritation, fatigue, and breast tissue changes, which can occur during or shortly after treatment.
 Furthermore, the long-term effects, including the risk of developing secondary cancers in the radiation-exposed area, should be conveyed. While emphasizing these risks, it's crucial to underscore that advances in radiation therapy techniques have significantly minimized the chances of long-term effects, and close collaboration with healthcare teams can effectively manage potential side effects.

.

Navigating Decisions:

Empowering readers to navigate decisions about radiation therapy involves presenting a balanced view of its benefits and risks. Understanding the significance of individualized treatment planning and the incorporation of patient preferences is key.
 Moreover, highlighting the collaborative nature of the decision-making process between patients and their healthcare providers fosters a sense of agency and confidence. By emphasizing the importance of open communication and shared decision-making, patients are encouraged to actively engage in their treatment planning process, ensuring that their preferences and values are duly considered.

In essence, providing an articulate and engaging exploration of radiation therapy's benefits and risks enriches readers' understanding of this pivotal treatment modality. Equipped with comprehensive knowledge, they are better prepared to approach treatment decisions with confidence and actively participate in their care. This nuanced understanding fosters a sense of empowerment, resilience, and informed engagement with their healthcare providers, thereby contributing to a more holistic and patient-centered treatment experience.

Targeted therapy and immunotherapy have emerged as revolutionary frontiers in the fight against cancer, showcasing remarkable potential in addressing breast cancer and other malignancies. By illuminating the distinctive features of these treatments, we can grasp their transformative impact on patient care and prognosis.

Targeted Therapy:

 We are introduced to the concept of targeted therapy, which involves the use of drugs or other substances to precisely identify and attack cancer cells. In the context of breast cancer, targeted therapy often focuses on specific molecules or pathways within cancer cells that drive their growth and spread. By honing in on these specific targets, targeted therapy seeks to disrupt the cancer cells' ability to proliferate, thereby impeding tumor growth and metastasis. Notably, you should be informed about the various targeted therapies available for different subtypes of breast cancer, underscoring the increasingly personalized nature of cancer treatment.

Immunotherapy:

Immunotherapy, harnessing the body's immune system to combat cancer, represents a paradigm shift in cancer treatment. We are introduced to the concept of immune checkpoint inhibitors, which help unleash the immune system to recognize and attack cancer cells. In the landscape of breast cancer, ongoing research endeavors to unravel the potential of immunotherapy, particularly in certain subtypes of the disease. By highlighting the principles and potential limitations of immunotherapy, we can appreciate the evolving role of this innovative approach and remain informed about breakthroughs in the field.

Combined Potential:

Exploring the synergistic potential of targeted therapy and immunotherapy piques your interest and underscores the multifaceted nature of modern cancer treatment. Recent research suggests that combining these modalities may lead to enhanced treatment outcomes, offering a glimpse into the future of combination therapies for breast cancer. By emphasizing the promise of combined approaches, we are encouraged to consider the rapidly evolving treatment landscape and the potential for increasingly tailored and effective therapeutic regimens.

In conclusion, by offering an insightful and persuasive overview of targeted therapy and immunotherapy, we are equipped with a profound understanding of these groundbreaking treatments. This knowledge empowers us to engage in informed discussions with healthcare providers, stay abreast of emerging treatment options, and make informed decisions about care. As advocates for their own health, patients are primed to embrace the promise of targeted therapy and immunotherapy while remaining cognizant of their evolving role in shaping the future of cancer treatment.

Chapter 4: Integrative Approaches to Healing

4.1 Complementary and Alternative Medicine.

Integrative Approaches to Healing commences with an exploration of complementary and alternative medicine (CAM), offering you a comprehensive view of these diverse and holistic therapeutic modalities.
CAM encompasses a spectrum of practices and approaches that diverge from conventional Western medicine, aiming to complement or serve as alternatives to traditional treatments. By shedding light on this multifaceted landscape, readers can glean insights into the rich tapestry of healing modalities available to them.

Complementary Medicine:

Complementary medicine encompasses practices and interventions that are used alongside conventional medical treatments. These may include acupuncture, herbal remedies, yoga, massage therapy, and dietary supplements, among others.
By bolstering conventional care, complementary medicine endeavors to enhance overall well-being, alleviate treatment side effects, and foster a sense of holistic balance.

Alternative Medicine:

Alternative medicine, in contrast, encapsulates therapies often used in lieu of conventional medical treatments. These may encompass traditional Chinese medicine, naturopathy, Ayurveda, and homeopathy, among others. While recognizing the autonomy and diverse perspectives of individuals opting for alternative medicine, it's crucial to present a nuanced view, emphasizing the importance of evidence-based decision-making and the potential risks associated with solely relying on alternative modalities for the treatment of serious medical conditions.

Navigating Choices for Healing:

Empowering readers to navigate the realms of complementary and alternative medicine involves fostering informed decision-making and a comprehensive understanding of these modalities. By emphasizing the significance of open communication with healthcare providers, we are encouraged to participate actively in their treatment plans, ensuring that integrative approaches are harmoniously integrated within the framework of evidence-based care. Moreover, an exploration of the potential benefits and limitations of these modalities offers readers a balanced perspective and encourages them to approach these therapies with discernment and awareness.

4.2 Mind-body Techniques : Meditation, Yoga and Visualization.

Integrative Approaches to Healing explores further into the intricate tapestry of mind-body techniques, encapsulating the transformative potential of meditation, yoga, and visualization in fostering holistic well-being. By illuminating the profound impact of these practices, we are made to embark on a journey of self-discovery and empowerment, cultivating an enriching understanding of the interconnectedness between mind, body, and spirit.

Meditation:

Meditation serves as a foundational pillar in the domain of mind-body techniques, offering individuals a pathway to inner tranquility and self-awareness. By acquainting readers with diverse forms of meditation, including mindfulness meditation, loving-kindness meditation, and transcendental meditation, they gain insight into the multifaceted nature of this practice. Furthermore, elucidating the scientific underpinnings of meditation equips readers with a deeper comprehension of its potential benefits, ranging from stress reduction and emotional regulation to enhancing cognitive function and fostering resilience in the face of adversity.

Yoga:

Yoga, an ancient practice steeped in tradition, emerges as a dynamic fusion of physical postures, breathwork, and meditation. Going up into the multifaceted dimensions of yoga, readers embark on a journey to explore its therapeutic potential in promoting physical strength, flexibility, and balance, while simultaneously nurturing mental serenity and emotional equilibrium. By emphasizing the varied styles of yoga, such as Hatha, Vinyasa, and Kundalini, readers gain an appreciation for the diverse pathways to harnessing the transformative power of this venerable practice.

Visualization:

Visualization, a captivating tool for harnessing the mind's creative potential, emerges as a compelling avenue for us to explore the intersection of imagination and healing. By illuminating the principles of creative visualization and guided imagery, readers are invited to embark on an inward odyssey, tapping into the profound ability of the mind to shape one's reality and cultivate a profound sense of well-being. Notably, visualization plays an integral role in supporting individuals through challenging medical treatments, fostering resilience, and serving as a catalyst for inner healing and renewal.

Crafting an in-depth exploration of these mind-body techniques enriches readers' understanding of the profound interconnectedness between mental, emotional, and physical well-being. By fostering a nuanced appreciation for the transformative potential of meditation, yoga, and visualization, readers are empowered to embrace these practices as integral components of their holistic well-being journey, nurturing a profound sense of balance, resilience, and inner harmony.

Ultimately, providing an engaging and authentic exploration of complementary and alternative medicine enriches readers' understanding of the myriad options available for healing. By fostering a well-rounded appreciation of these integrative modalities, you are empowered to make informed decisions about health, actively engage with healthcare providers, and craft personalized treatment journeys that resonate with their values and aspirations for holistic well-being.

4.3 Supportive Therapies: Acupuncture Massage and Reiki.

In the pursuit of holistic well-being, individuals often seek solace and relief through supportive therapies that encompass acupuncture, massage, and Reiki, embodying diverse modalities that resonate with the intricacies of the human experience. Tailoring the discussion to address the needs of individuals in search of guidance, comfort, and effective therapeutic interventions, the exploration of supportive therapies navigates the transformative potential inherent in these age-old practices.

Acupuncture:

Individuals seeking holistic healing and relief from a spectrum of physical and emotional ailments often gravitate towards acupuncture, an ancient tradition rooted in the principles of traditional Chinese medicine. By acknowledging the vitality of the body's energy pathways, or meridians, acupuncture offers individuals a pathway to harmony and vitality. Addressing the potential of acupuncture to alleviate pain, mitigate stress, and restore balance, readers gain a nuanced understanding of this therapeutic artistry, fostering a sense of hope and empowerment in their quest for healing.

Massage:

The profound art of massage emerges as a beacon of comfort and rejuvenation, embracing a diverse array of modalities that speak to the intricate needs of individuals. Whether seeking relief from muscular tension, stress, or simply desiring a sanctum of tranquility, massage embodies an oasis of healing. By illustrating the diverse styles of massage, including

Swedish, deep tissue, and aromatherapy massage, readers are invited to embrace the transformative potential of touch, recognizing its capacity to nurture the body, soothe the spirit, and foster a profound sense of well-being.

Reiki:

Embarking on a spiritual odyssey, individuals yearning for holistic healing often find solace in the timeless practice of Reiki, which revolves around the channeling of universal life energy to restore balance and vitality. Gently guiding readers through the nuances of Reiki, they are beckoned into a realm of subtle energy work, inviting contemplation and renewal. By emphasizing the potential of Reiki to enhance relaxation, facilitate emotional healing, and reinvigorate the spirit, readers embolden their quest for serenity and inner healing.

By nurturing a profound understanding of these supportive therapies, readers are extended an empathetic embrace, empowering them in their journey towards holistic well-being. By honoring the diverse needs and aspirations of individuals, this exploration illuminates the transformative potential inherent in acupuncture, massage, and Reiki, inspiring hope, resilience, and a profound sense of connectedness to the healing journey.

4.4 Creating a Holistic Recovery Plan

In the pursuit of comprehensive well-being, the endeavor to craft a holistic recovery plan encapsulates an intricate tapestry of considerations, aspirations, and integrative modalities that resonate with the unique journey of each individual. Embracing a compassionate lens that acknowledges the complexities and nuances of personal healing, the exploration of creating a holistic recovery plan becomes a poignant odyssey, inviting individuals to embrace the transformative power inherent in this multifaceted endeavor.

Identifying Individual Needs:

Embarking on the quest for holistic recovery involves an introspective odyssey, one that beckons individuals to engage with their deepest aspirations, challenges, and aspirations. By fostering a compassionate understanding of individual needs, aspirations, and challenges, the process of crafting a holistic recovery plan becomes an act of self-empowerment, one that invites individuals to cultivate a profound sense of agency, authenticity, and self-awareness.

Integrating Diverse Modalities:

Addressing the multifaceted dimensions of holistic recovery extends beyond conventional paradigms, encompassing a rich mosaic of integrative modalities that speak to the interconnectedness of mind, body, and spirit. By fostering an inclusive environment that celebrates diversity, the process of integrating diverse modalities, such as nutrition, exercise, mindfulness practices, and therapeutic interventions, unfolds as a symphony of adaptive healing tailored to the unique needs and aspirations of each individual.

Nurturing Emotional Well-being:

The terrain of holistic recovery embraces the emotive landscape of the human experience, offering individuals a sanctuary to nourish emotional well-being, navigate transformative experiences, and foster resilience. By fostering an environment that reveres emotional authenticity, the holistic recovery plan becomes a catalyst for nurturing emotional well-being, providing individuals with the space to explore mindfulness practices, counseling, expressive arts therapies, and other modalities that foster emotional equilibrium and inner harmony.

Cultivating Supportive Networks:

The quest for holistic recovery unfolds within the tapestry of supportive networks, honoring the interconnectedness of individuals with their communities, loved ones, and healthcare providers. By fostering an empathetic environment that values the significance of supportive networks, individuals are encouraged to seek solace in support groups, cultivate open communication with healthcare providers, and lean on the pillars of community and familial support, illuminating the transformative potential of collective empathy and understanding.

Crafting a holistic recovery plan embodies an intimate odyssey, one that resonates with the intricate web of individual experiences, aspirations, and transformative potential. By nurturing an environment that honors the multifaceted dimensions of holistic recovery, individuals engage in a profound act of self-discovery, resilience, and empowerment, fostering a sense of agency and hope as they navigate the transformative landscape of their well-being journey.

Chapter 5 Navigating Emotional and Mental Health.

5.1 Coping with Diagnosis and Treatment.

Navigating the emotional and mental terrain following a diagnosis and during treatment comprises a transformative odyssey, one that necessitates profound resilience, adaptive coping mechanisms, and an unwavering commitment to holistic well-being. To make this process a success in a relatively short time frame, individuals can embrace several strategies and perspectives:

1. **Cultivating Emotional Resilience**:
Embracing the emotional nuances of a diagnosis and treatment involves cultivating emotional resilience, encouraging individuals to acknowledge and process their emotions authentically. By fostering a compassionate understanding of one's emotional landscape, individuals can engage in practices such as journaling, mindfulness, or seeking the support of a mental health professional.

2. **Seeking Knowledge and Support:**
Rapidly navigating the complexities of a diagnosis and treatment process entails seeking knowledge and support from reputable sources. By empowering oneself

with accurate information, individuals can engage in open and informed dialogue with healthcare providers, actively participate in decision-making, and seek the solace of support groups or trusted loved ones.

3. **Embracing Self-care Practices:**

Amidst the rigors of diagnosis and treatment, individuals can expedite their success by embracing self-care practices that nurture their physical, emotional, and mental well-being. Incorporating activities such as gentle exercise, adequate rest, nourishing meals, and engaging in activities that bring joy and relaxation can infuse vitality and resilience into their journey.

4. **Emphasizing Open Communication:**

Creating a success-oriented trajectory involves emphasizing open and honest communication with healthcare providers, loved ones, and support networks. By fostering a candid dialogue, individuals can voice their needs, concerns, and aspirations, thus fortifying a network of understanding and empathy that contributes to their overall well-being.

5. **Fostering a Sense of Purpose and Meaning:**

Navigating the landscape of a diagnosis and treatment process expeditiously involves nurturing a profound sense of purpose and meaning. Engaging in activities that resonate with personal passions, exploring creative pursuits, or finding ways to contribute to others can imbue the journey with a sense of empowerment and inspiration.

By embracing these diverse strategies and perspectives, individuals can expedite their success in coping with diagnosis and treatment, fostering a resilient and transformative trajectory conducive to holistic well-being and emotional equilibrium.

5.2. Building a Strong Support Network.

Building a robust support network during trying times is fundamental to nurturing emotional and mental well-being. Research has consistently shown that strong social support is linked to better mental health outcomes (Cohen, 2004). Below are practical steps to build a supportive network:

1. **Identify Trusted Individuals**:
Start by identifying individuals in your life whom you trust and feel comfortable confiding in. This may include family members, close friends, mentors, or colleagues who have shown empathy and understanding.

2. **Seek Peer Support:**
Consider joining support groups or communities comprising individuals who have gone through similar

.

experiences. This can provide a sense of belonging, shared understanding, and valuable insights (Al-Abri & Al-Balushi, 2014).

3. **Communicate Your Needs:**
Open and honest communication is crucial. Clearly communicate your needs, whether it's a listening ear, practical assistance, or emotional support. This fosters an environment of understanding and empathy (House, 1981).

4. **Diversify Your Network**:
Consciously diversify your support network to include individuals with varied perspectives, interests, and experiences. This can offer a broader range of insights and support, enriching your overall experience (Lakey & Heller, 2016).

5. **Professional Support**:
Seeking guidance from mental health professionals or counselors can provide a structured, therapeutic form of support. Their expertise can complement and enhance the support received from friends and family (Fox, 2002).

6. **Reciprocity and Gratitude**:
In nurturing your support network, remember to reciprocate the support you receive and express gratitude. Engaging in acts of kindness and offering

support in return can further strengthen your bonds with others (Sbarra & Hazan, 2008).

7. Community Resources:

Explore local or online resources, such as community centers, helplines, or religious organizations, which may offer additional forms of support, guidance, or group activities.

By actively engaging in the process of building a robust support network, individuals can fortify their emotional resilience and enhance their capacity to navigate the challenges of life with a greater sense of connectedness and well-being.

.

5.3. Mental Health Resources and Counselling.

Mental health resources and counseling play a pivotal role in the treatment and recovery processes, offering essential support and guidance to individuals navigating the complexities of mental health challenges. Here are the key ways in which these resources contribute to the treatment and recovery journeys:

.

1. **Access to Expertise and Support**:
Mental health resources and counseling provide
individuals with access to the expertise of trained
professionals, including psychologists, counselors, and
therapists. These professionals offer a safe,
non-judgmental space where individuals can express
their emotions, discuss challenges, and receive
guidance tailored to their unique needs.

2. **Therapeutic Interventions:**
Counseling and mental health resources encompass a
diverse range of therapeutic interventions, including
cognitive-behavioral therapy (CBT), dialectical behavior
therapy (DBT), and mindfulness-based approaches.
These interventions equip individuals with valuable
coping skills, emotional regulation techniques, and
strategies to navigate their mental health challenges
effectively.

3. **Holistic Treatment Approach**:
Mental health resources and counseling often embrace
a holistic treatment approach that recognizes the
interconnectedness of mental, emotional, and physical
well-being. By addressing the individual as a whole,
these resources aim to foster comprehensive healing
and empower individuals to lead fulfilling lives.

4. **Education and Empowerment:**
Through counseling and mental health resources,
individuals receive education about their mental health

conditions, gaining a deeper understanding of their challenges and potential paths to recovery. This knowledge empowers individuals to actively participate in their treatment journey and make informed decisions regarding their well-being.

5. Coping Strategies and Support Network Enhancement:

Counseling sessions provide a platform to develop and refine effective coping strategies to manage stress, anxiety, depression, or other mental health concerns. Additionally, mental health resources can aid in enhancing an individual's support network by connecting them with peer groups, community resources, and other avenues of support.

6. Long-Term Recovery Maintenance:

Mental health resources and counseling are instrumental in supporting individuals not only through the initial stages of treatment but also in maintaining long-term recovery. Regular counseling sessions, support groups, and access to mental health resources form a continuum of care that promotes sustained well-being and resilience.

In conclusion, mental health resources and counseling form an integral part of the treatment and recovery processes, offering a multifaceted approach to addressing mental health challenges, fostering resilience, and empowering individuals on their journey toward holistic well-being.

5.4. Addressing Fear and Anxiety

Addressing fear and anxiety during the diagnosis and treatment period is crucial for maintaining emotional well-being and overall resilience. Here are some profitable ways to overcome these challenges:

1. **Knowledge Is Power**:
Empowerment through knowledge is an effective way to alleviate fear and anxiety. Learning about the diagnosis, treatment options, and potential outcomes from reputable sources can provide clarity and reduce uncertainty, empowering individuals to actively participate in their care.

2. **Cultivate Mindfulness and Relaxation:**
Practicing mindfulness, deep breathing, meditation, or yoga can significantly reduce anxiety and promote a sense of calm. These relaxation techniques help individuals stay grounded and cope with the emotional

turbulence that accompanies the diagnosis and treatment process.

3. **Seek Emotional Support:**
Sharing fears and anxieties with trusted loved ones, support groups, or mental health professionals can provide immense relief. Expressing emotions openly can help individuals feel understood, supported, and less isolated in their experiences.

4. **Engage in Distractions and Hobbies**:
Immersing oneself in enjoyable activities and hobbies can act as a powerful distraction from fears and anxieties. Engaging in creative outlets, physical activities, or hobbies can provide moments of respite and positive reinforcement.

5. **Maintain Open Communication with Healthcare Providers:**
Openly discussing fears and anxieties with healthcare providers encourages candid conversations about concerns and potential solutions. This fosters a collaborative approach to care and can alleviate fears stemming from uncertainty.

6. **Set Realistic Goals and Celebrate Small Victories:**
Setting achievable, short-term goals can instill a sense of achievement and progress, countering feelings of helplessness and fear. Celebrating small victories, no

matter how insignificant they may seem, reinforces
resilience and positivity.

7. **Embrace Supportive Literature and Media:**
Exploring literature, podcasts, or films that emphasize
hope, resilience, and the triumph of the human spirit can
inspire and uplift individuals facing fear and anxiety.
Positive narratives can instill a sense of optimism and
strength.

By embracing these profitable strategies, individuals can
navigate the diagnosis and treatment period with
resilience, effectively manage fear and anxiety, and lay a
foundation for emotional well-being during this
challenging time.

Chapter 6: Life After Treatment

6.1 Survivorship: Embracing A New Normal

Survivorship marks the beginning of a new chapter in the lives of individuals who have completed their treatment for a serious illness. Embracing this "new normal" involves navigating various physical, emotional, and social changes while striving to lead a fulfilling life. Here are some key points to consider during this phase:

1. **Physical Recovery and Rehabilitation:**
After treatment, individuals may experience physical changes, including fatigue, reduced stamina, or lingering side effects. Engaging in tailored rehabilitation programs, such as physical therapy or supervised exercise, can aid in restoring physical function and enhancing overall well-being.

2. **Emotional Well-being and Coping Strategies:**
Adjusting to life after treatment involves addressing emotional challenges, such as anxiety, fear of recurrence, or post-treatment depression. Seeking counseling, support groups, or individual therapy can help individuals develop coping strategies and manage the emotional impact of their survivorship.

3. **Managing Long-Term Side Effects**:
Some treatments may result in long-term side effects
that require ongoing management. It's essential for
individuals to maintain open communication with their
healthcare team, actively report any new symptoms, and
adhere to recommended follow-up care to address and
mitigate potential long-term effects.

4. **Reestablishing Social Connections:**
Survivorship often prompts a reevaluation of social
relationships and the reestablishment of meaningful
connections. Engaging in social activities, reconnecting
with friends and family, and seeking support from peer
groups or survivorship networks can aid in rebuilding a
robust social support system.

5. **Redefining Personal Goals and Priorities:**
This phase offers an opportunity for individuals to reflect
on their values, goals, and aspirations, potentially
leading to a redefinition of personal priorities. Exploring
new interests, setting achievable goals, and pursuing
meaningful endeavors contribute to a sense of purpose
and reinvigorate life post-treatment.

6. **Celebrating Milestones and Acknowledging
Resilience**:
Acknowledging and celebrating milestones, whether big
or small, is vital in recognizing personal resilience and
strength. Reflecting on the journey from diagnosis to

survivorship reinforces an individual's determination and fortitude.

7. **Advocacy and Giving Back:**
Many survivors find a sense of fulfillment in advocating for others facing similar challenges. Becoming involved in advocacy, mentoring, or supporting charitable initiatives can provide a deeper purpose and positively impact others within the survivorship community.

Overall, survivorship represents an opportunity for individuals to embrace a new normal, redefine their paths, and cultivate resilience as they navigate life beyond treatment. By addressing physical, emotional, and social dimensions, individuals can lay the groundwork for a fulfilling and empowered survivorship journey.

6.2 Follow-up Care and Monitoring: The Key to Long-term Success

Follow-up care and monitoring are crucial elements in ensuring the success of any endeavor, and this is especially true in the realm of healthcare. Whether it's post-operative care, chronic disease itmanagement, or simply maintaining overall wellness, regular follow-up and monitoring play a vital role in ensuring positive outcomes and preventing potential complications.

One of the most profitable attitudes to adopt when it comes to follow-up care and monitoring is a proactive and patient-centered approach.
 This means going beyond the mere fulfillment of routine check-ups and appointments, and instead, actively engaging with patients to understand their unique needs and concerns. By taking the time to listen and empathize with patients, healthcare providers can build trust and rapport, ultimately leading to better adherence to treatment plans and improved health outcomes.

In addition to a patient-centered approach, a commitment to ongoing education and communication is essential for effective follow-up care and monitoring. This involves not only providing patients with clear and comprehensive information about their condition and treatment plan but also empowering them to take an active role in their own care. By fostering open lines of communication and encouraging patients to ask questions and voice their concerns, healthcare providers can ensure that follow-up care is truly tailored to the individual needs of each patient.

Furthermore, embracing a multidisciplinary approach to follow-up care and monitoring can significantly enhance its effectiveness. By involving a diverse team of healthcare professionals, including nurses, pharmacists, nutritionists, and mental health specialists, patients can benefit from a comprehensive and holistic approach to their care. This not only ensures that all aspects of their health are being addressed but also allows for early intervention and personalized support when needed.

Finally, a commitment to leveraging technology and data-driven insights can greatly enhance the quality of follow-up care and monitoring. From remote monitoring devices to electronic health records, healthcare providers can harness the power of technology to track patient progress, identify potential issues early on, and tailor interventions based on real-time data.

In conclusion, by adopting a proactive, patient-centered approach, committing to ongoing education and communication, embracing a multidisciplinary team-based approach, and leveraging technology and data-driven insights, healthcare providers can ensure that follow-up care and monitoring is not only profitable in terms of improved patient outcomes but also fulfilling in terms of building meaningful patient-provider relationships.

6.3. Reclaiming Confidence and Body Image

Reclaiming confidence and body image after a traumatic event or illness is a deeply personal journey, but it is one that can be achieved with the right support and mindset. Survivors often face physical and emotional challenges that can impact their self-esteem and how they perceive their bodies. However, there are several strategies that can help survivors reclaim their confidence and improve their body image.

First and foremost, it's important for survivors to practice self-compassion and patience. Healing takes time, and it's okay to have moments of vulnerability. Seeking support from friends, family, or a therapist can provide a safe space to process emotions and work through any negative feelings about their bodies.

Engaging in activities that promote self-care and self-expression can also be empowering. This could include practicing yoga, meditation, or engaging in creative outlets such as art or writing. These activities can help survivors reconnect with their bodies in a positive way and build a sense of inner strength.

Another key aspect of reclaiming confidence and body image is finding a supportive community. Connecting with other survivors who have gone through similar experiences can provide a sense of solidarity and understanding. Support groups or online communities can offer valuable encouragement and inspiration, reminding survivors that they are not alone in their journey.

Additionally, focusing on overall health and well-being, rather than solely on appearance, can shift the focus away from negative body image. Engaging in regular physical activity, eating nourishing foods, and getting enough rest can all contribute to a positive sense of self-worth and confidence.

Finally, practicing positive affirmations and challenging negative self-talk can help survivors reframe their thoughts about their bodies. By consciously shifting the internal dialogue to focus on strengths and resilience, survivors can gradually cultivate a more positive body image and regain confidence.

In conclusion, reclaiming confidence and body image is an ongoing process that requires patience, self-care, support from others, and a shift in mindset. By embracing these strategies, survivors can take significant steps toward rebuilding their confidence and embracing a positive body image.

6.4 Long-term Health and Wellness Strategies.

One unique and simple long-term health and wellness strategy is the practice of mindful movement. This approach focuses on integrating physical activity with mindfulness techniques to promote overall well-being. Mindful movement encompasses various activities such as yoga, tai chi, qigong, and even walking or running with a focus on being present in the moment.

Engaging in mindful movement not only promotes physical health but also supports mental and emotional well-being. By incorporating mindfulness into physical activity, individuals can cultivate a deeper connection between their bodies and minds, leading to a more holistic approach to health and wellness.

One of the key benefits of mindful movement is its ability to reduce stress and promote relaxation. Mindfulness techniques such as deep breathing, body awareness, and focused attention help individuals to release tension and calm the mind, which can have a positive impact on overall health.

Furthermore, mindful movement encourages individuals to listen to their bodies and honor their physical limitations. This approach emphasizes self-compassion and self-care, allowing individuals to engage in physical activity without pushing themselves beyond their capabilities, thus reducing the risk of injury and burnout.

In addition, mindful movement can improve flexibility, balance, and posture, leading to better physical function and reduced risk of musculoskeletal issues as individuals age. The gentle, deliberate movements characteristic of mindful practices can also be accessible to people of varying fitness levels and ages, making it an inclusive long-term health strategy.

Moreover, the mind-body connection fostered by mindful movement can lead to greater body awareness and acceptance. Over time, individuals may develop a more positive body image and a deeper appreciation for what their bodies can achieve, contributing to enhanced self-esteem and overall well-being.

In summary, incorporating mindful movement into daily life can serve as a unique and simple long-term health and wellness strategy. By combining physical activity with mindfulness techniques, individuals can experience a wide range of benefits that support their long-term health, both physically and emotionally.

Chapter 7. Empowerment and Advocacy

7.1 Overcoming Stigma and Misconceptions

Education, awareness, and open discussions are key components in addressing stigma and misconceptions surrounding breast cancer.

Education about breast cancer, its risk factors, symptoms, and treatment options, can help dispel myths and reduce stigma. Public campaigns, community workshops, and school programs can provide accurate information about breast cancer, encouraging individuals to seek early detection and treatment.

Media portrayal of breast cancer also plays a significant role in shaping public perceptions. Responsible reporting on breast cancer can help challenge stereotypes and reduce stigma. Journalists and media professionals should be encouraged to portray breast cancer topics accurately and sensitively.

Open discussions about breast cancer can help break down barriers and reduce stigma. Encouraging individuals to share their experiences and challenges can foster empathy and understanding in the community. Support groups and peer-led initiatives provide safe spaces for individuals to connect with others who have been affected by breast cancer, reducing feelings of isolation and shame.

Advocacy efforts are crucial in addressing systemic stigma and discrimination related to breast cancer. Advocacy involves speaking out against injustices and promoting policies that protect the rights of individuals affected by breast cancer. By advocating for increased access to screening, treatment, and support services, advocates can create a more inclusive and supportive environment for those affected by breast cancer.

In conclusion, overcoming stigma and misconceptions surrounding breast cancer is essential for empowering individuals and advocating for their rights. By promoting education, responsible media portrayal, open discussions, and advocacy efforts, society can work towards creating a more supportive and understanding environment for individuals affected by breast cancer.

7.2 Advocacy For Policy changes and Funding.

Advocacy for policy changes and funding is a critical component in the fight against breast cancer. It is a call to action, a passionate plea to lawmakers and decision-makers to prioritize the needs of those affected by breast cancer and allocate resources to support research, prevention, and treatment. This advocacy is not just a matter of raising awareness; it is a powerful force that drives real, tangible change.

By advocating for policy changes, individuals and organizations can push for legislation that ensures access to affordable and comprehensive healthcare for all individuals, regardless of their socioeconomic status. This includes advocating for policies that guarantee coverage for essential breast cancer screenings, diagnostic tests, and treatments, as well as supporting initiatives that address health disparities and inequities in access to care.

Advocacy for funding is equally crucial, as it fuels groundbreaking research and innovative treatments. It involves rallying support for increased investment in breast cancer research, which can lead to the development of more effective therapies and ultimately save lives. Advocates also work to secure funding for support services, such as patient navigation programs, counseling, and survivorship programs, which are vital in providing comprehensive care to individuals facing a breast cancer diagnosis.

Furthermore, advocacy for policy changes and funding extends beyond the realm of healthcare. It encompasses efforts to promote workplace policies that support individuals undergoing treatment, such as paid leave and reasonable accommodations. It also involves advocating for environmental policies that address potential carcinogens and promote healthy living environments.

In essence, advocacy for policy changes and funding is a resounding call to action, urging policymakers to prioritize the fight against breast cancer. It is a relentless pursuit of equity, access, and progress in the quest to eradicate this disease. Through unwavering advocacy efforts, we can drive meaningful change, improve outcomes for those affected by breast cancer, and ultimately move closer to a world free from the burden of this devastating illness.

7.3 Inspiring Stories of Triumph and Resilience.

Title: Finding Strength in the Battle Against Breast
Cancer

As I sat in the waiting room, the ticking of the clock
seemed to mimic the turmoil in my mind. The diagnosis
had hit me like a sledgehammer, leaving me stumbling
in a whirlwind of fear and uncertainty. It was at that
moment, amidst the chaos, that I wished for a beacon of
hope to guide me through the challenging journey
ahead.

In a room filled with apprehension, I met Sarah, a breast
cancer survivor whose radiance was a testament to her
resilience. Her story unfolded like a delicate tapestry,
woven with threads of courage, vulnerability, and
unwavering hope. She shared her insights, emphasizing
the importance of self-care and the power of a
supportive community. Her practical advice turned mere
words into life-saving wisdom, providing a roadmap for
navigating the complexities of treatment and recovery.

As I got deeper into the labyrinth of uncertainty, I
encountered Dr. Jones, an oncologist whose
compassion shone through her every action. Her gentle
demeanor and wealth of knowledge became my pillars
of strength. Dr. Jones offered me a holistic perspective,

.

emphasizing the significance of mental well-being alongside medical treatment. Her guidance illuminated the path forward, helping me uncover the resilience that resided within me.

These real-life narratives of hope and triumph echo the sentiment that, in the face of adversity, the human spirit is indomitable. They reinforce the notion that while the road ahead may be fraught with challenges, it is also lined with opportunities for growth, empathy, and unwavering strength.

Through the shared experiences of survivors and healthcare professionals, I discovered that the journey through breast cancer is indeed a formidable one, but it is also a testament to the unyielding human spirit and the boundless power of hope.

Conclusion

"Conquering Breast Cancer: A Guide to Prevention and Recovery", is a book that serves as a beacon of knowledge and empowerment for individuals facing the challenges of breast cancer.

This comprehensive resource has provided valuable insights into prevention strategies, early detection methods, treatment options, and holistic approaches to recovery. By delving into the pages of this book, readers have gained a deeper understanding of the complexities of breast cancer and have been equipped with the tools to make informed decisions about their health.

As we close this chapter, let us remember that knowledge is power. Armed with the information and guidance from this book, we are better prepared to confront this disease with resilience and hope. It is a call to action for all individuals to prioritize their breast health, advocate for regular screenings, and seek support from healthcare professionals and support networks.

Let us stand together in solidarity, spreading awareness and promoting proactive measures for breast cancer prevention. Whether you are a survivor, a caregiver, or an advocate, let the knowledge gained from this book propel you into action. Let us continue to support ongoing research, promote early detection, and provide unwavering support to those affected by breast cancer.

Together, we can make a difference in the fight against breast cancer. Let us carry the wisdom and encouragement from "Conquering Breast Cancer" forward, as we strive to create a world free from the burden of this disease.

Resources and References

Support Organizations:
1. Susan G. Komen: A leading organization dedicated to breast cancer research, education, and support services for patients and their families. Their website offers a wealth of resources, including information on treatment options, support groups, and survivorship programs.

2. National Breast Cancer Foundation: This organization provides comprehensive support for individuals affected by breast cancer, offering resources such as financial assistance for treatment, early detection programs, and educational materials on breast health.

Websites:
1. Breastcancer.org: An extensive online platform offering evidence-based information on breast cancer prevention, diagnosis, and treatment. The website features forums for peer support, expert-authored articles, and the latest research updates.

2. American Cancer Society: Their website provides a wealth of resources on breast cancer, including information on risk factors, screening guidelines, and support programs for patients and caregivers.

Recommended Books:
1. "The Breast Cancer Survival Manual" by John Link, MD: This comprehensive guide covers all aspects of

breast cancer diagnosis, treatment, and recovery, providing practical advice and emotional support for patients and their loved ones.

2. "Radical Remission: Surviving Cancer Against All Odds" by Kelly A. Turner, PhD: While not specifically focused on breast cancer, this book offers inspiring stories of individuals who have overcome cancer through unconventional means, providing hope and alternative perspectives on healing.

These resources offer invaluable support and insights for individuals seeking information on breast cancer prevention, treatment, and recovery. Whether accessing online platforms, seeking support from organizations, or delving into informative books, these references empower individuals to navigate the complexities of breast cancer with knowledge and resilience.

www.ingramcontent.com/pod-product-compliance
Lightning Source LLC
Chambersburg PA
CBHW070756250726
48662CB00004B/1833